Empath

The Complete Guide to Emotional, Psychological, and Spiritual Healing For Sensitive People

By: Mark Madison

Table of Contents

Introduction

Congratulations on downloading "*Empath*!"

As you read through this book, you will understand your gift of being an empath and feel a greater sense of empowerment when it comes to living your life and embracing your experiences here on Earth. As you read through it, you will gain the opportunity to fully understand what it means to be an empath (including from a psychological perspective) and identify all of the symptoms that you may be experiencing in your life. You will also have the opportunity to identify the importance of healing yourself and the many ways that you can do so in order to ensure that you can live your best life possible.

As an empath, healing gives you an exclusive opportunity to begin discovering why your sensitivities seem to have so much control over you and how you can take back control. It does not mean that you will stop being an empath; it does mean that you will have a greater sense of control over your ability to tune into the world around you. As a result, you will no longer feel as though you have to be completely plugged in all the time. This sense of control will support you in engaging in healthy detachment so that you can begin enjoying social experiences once more without feeling overwhelmed or overburdened by the energies around you.

Regardless of whether you are naturally introverted or naturally extroverted, having the capacity to go out and enjoy the public is an incredibly freeing experience. Most experiences will involve the public in one way or another, so allowing yourself to overcome these feelings of anxiety and overwhelm will support you in enjoying your experiences to a greater degree.

I encourage you to read this book slowly and to embrace each chapter one at a time. Once you enter the healing stages of the book, you might find that you have a lot to work through, especially if you are still living in the stage of your gift where you feel the energy around you to such a deep degree. Taking it slowly and giving yourself the time to embrace each step will ensure that you do not become overwhelmed or find yourself struggling to stay committed. If you are ready to take it easy and experience an incredibly powerful and insightful healing experience, it is time to begin! Please make sure to take your time and enjoy!

Chapter 1: The Empath Way

The term "empath" has recently become a popular topic in the spiritual community as people are now beginning to realize that being sensitive is a gift and that there is no reason to be ashamed of their empathic ways. As an empath, you possess a unique gift that provides you with the opportunity to genuinely feel the needs of others and the world and universe as a whole, allowing you to be a powerful healer of the world. Your gift provides you with the opportunity to sense where more love and compassion can be offered and then offer it as a way to contribute to the raising vibrations of this loving planet. However, if not used properly, being an empath can result in obsessive behaviors that deplete your energies and prevent you from experiencing the positive wonders of your gift.

If you know you are an empath or if you have a suspicion that you might be, you may have questions about what that means and where this gift even comes from. In this chapter, we are going to explore what it means to be an empath, why you are living with this gift, and how this gift can support you in living out your life's true purpose. We will begin with the history of what it means to be an empath and move through to a more modern definition to provide you with the opportunity to build your understanding of your gift and how it fits into the unique makeup of the universe.

The History of "Empath"

Over the past millennia, the term empath has risen up across many different religions and cultures as a way to describe people who were sensitive to others in a seemingly mystical way. In ancient African and First Nations tribes, empaths were considered gifted healers, philosophers, and spiritual teachers. They continue to be seen as such by these tribes which have been known to offer their empaths special blessings and compassionate treatment in exchange for having the empath share their gifts with the tribes. More recently, the phenomena have been popularized by psychologists who are interested in helping people across the globe understand their unique sensitivities and how they can master these sensitivities so they can thrive in life.

In recent history, Dr. Carl Rogers played an influential role in advancing the understanding of empathy and empathic gifts by suggesting that this may be a psycho or parapsychological phenomenon. Essentially, he believes that this is a unique way that certain people can understand another's perspective and support them in their lives. In his words, sometimes, just listening to someone else is not enough because what they truly need is empathy from others. Empaths, who are particularly gifted with empathy to the highest degree, are wonderful at offering this unique support to individuals.

Being an Empath in Today's World

Today, being an empath is quite different from how it has been for recognized empaths in the past. In certain tribes and communities, empaths were revered by their societies and offered immense amounts of support, compassion, and respect by those around them. For quite some time throughout Western cultures, however, people who experienced greater sensitivities than others were considered weak and were often shamed by their peers for their sensitive behaviors. As a result, society became quite grueling and uncomfortable for empaths, especially ones that had no idea they were empaths and found themselves feeling particularly vulnerable to their peers.

Over time, the understanding of what it means to be an empath has come to light and many empaths have been given the opportunity to explore their gifts with a greater understanding of what they are and why they experience them. This also offers empaths the opportunity to experience a greater sense of compassion towards themselves, as they are now capable of understanding that they are not weak at all. In fact, they are incredibly powerful and have the capacity to change the world as we know it by offering their loving, compassionate, and empathetic gifts into the collective and helping us raise the vibrational frequency of the whole planet.

As society continues shifting towards being one that is more compassionate towards its sensitive beings, empaths are being offered the opportunity to be met with a personal understanding of themselves as well as an understanding by their community. Rather than being so harshly penalized for their personality, many are now finding safe sanctuaries out in the world where they can engage in society and play an active role in their lives. The era of being a cursed empath who was considered weak is quickly coming to a close as empaths are now being understood and respected for their incredible gifts.

A Day in the Life of an Empath

If you are an empath, you might notice that your day-to-day life looks quite different from the lives of those around you. If you have yet to find a collective of people who understand what this feels like, it may still feel somewhat isolating and uncomfortable or even frustrating as you attempt to explain your experiences to others. This may be heightened by your current lack of understanding of how powerful you truly are and how you can actually harness your power to begin thriving in your life.

Chances are, when you wake up, you are instantly greeted with an immense amount of energy. You may find yourself literally "feeling" the energy of the day based on what day it is, which may or may not play into how you end up feeling throughout your morning. The experiences you have in the morning can significantly impact your energy, too. If they are positive, such as waking up and being greeted by your happy dog and enjoying dinner with your generally positive family, then your energies will likely feel whole and nourished. However, if you wake up to a home that is messy, a spouse that experiences morning grumpiness or a sad child who had a nightmare, you may find yourself instantly being greeted with fairly intense energies that are matching the energies of those around you. This can be challenging when you are attempting to face your day with a positive energy but instead, find yourself feeling overwhelmed and even drained before the day has even really begun.

If you work or spend your day alongside other people, the bulk of your work day may feel overwhelming, as you are constantly taking on these energies and feeling them as if they were your own. For example, if someone comes into work late and everyone is cranky because it has slowed down the workflow, you may find yourself feeling cranky and exhausted, as well because you are taking on the crankiness of both yourself and everyone else. If you are fortunate enough to spend your days working in a positive environment, you may find yourself feeling exceptionally positive throughout the day, but still feeling particularly drained after work because of how many different kinds of energy you have embraced.

Once you return home, you may find yourself feeling exhausted and depleted. Whether or not your day was positive, the amount of energy it took to experience and feel all of the energies around you was probably overwhelming and left you feeling like you had nothing left for yourself. You may spend your evenings laying low and doing next to nothing as a way to try and relax and let your energy replenish so that you can do it again the next day.

If this day to day flow resonates with you, then you are experiencing the life of an empath who has not yet fully understood, accepted, and mastered their empathic gifts. As you read through the rest of this book, you will discover that your life does not have to feel like this at all and that you can most definitely experience a more positive and enjoyable life without feeling depleted at the end of every day. In fact, you will begin to discover how you can have more energy for yourself so that you can truly get the most out of life while still being masterfully talented with your empathic gift!

The Empath Calling

Being particularly sensitive to the energy of others means that you were born with an incredible gift that can truly help you change the world. You are the very person that is needed in order to help overcome the collective suffering that has been experienced for hundreds of years through wars, greed, and ignorance. Through your ability to experience complete empathy to such a deep degree, you can genuinely listen to and understand people and support them in their healing journeys. When someone needs to experience love, compassion, guidance, or reassurance, they know that they can come to you and experience that. Since this is what the world greatly lacks right now, this makes you the perfect person to offer it to the world.

Chances are, you have already seen this trend in your life with the immense amount of people who have looked to you for support or compassion. In fact, this pattern may have become so intense that you find yourself withdrawing and avoiding relationships because sometimes, it may feel like they require more energy than you have left. This may lead to feelings of guilt or even loneliness in your life, but to you that may seem like a reasonable price to pay to avoid feeling overburdened by the energy of yourself and everyone else around you.

Empaths often find themselves being called into positions of healers, caretakers, advocates, and teachers. This is because they possess the unique characteristics required to truly succeed in these fields and make a genuine difference in the world around them. However, left unmanaged, their empathic gifts may lead to them feeling overwhelmed and unable to pursue these callings for fear of being zapped of energy and constantly drained. If they learn to master their gift and use their empathic talents to their benefit, though, they will find that by pursuing these roles and fully stepping into them, they can genuinely make massive changes in the world around them.

Some of the most influential leaders, healers, and teachers of our time are known to be empaths. Oprah Winfrey, Deepak Chopra, Princess Diana, the Dalai Lama, and Mahatma Gandhi are all famous empaths who have stepped into their roles, mastered them, and fulfilled their purposes in life. This proves that it can be done and it can be done in a magnificent way so long as you take the time to genuinely understand yourself, have compassion for yourself, and fulfill your own needs as an empath and as a human.

A Realistic Understanding

Realizing that your purpose in life is to heal the world may come across as intense, overwhelming or even shocking. On one hand, you may find that it makes complete sense given your nature and the way that you naturally interact with those around you combined with your innate calling. On the other hand, taking on that large of a task may seem daunting and even impossible if you do not take the time to see it realistically and put it into perspective.

To help you feel a little less intimidated by your purpose, I want to remind you that you *are not alone.* You are not the only empath that exists, and you are not the only empath who possesses the purpose of supporting the collective in healing so that we can raise our collective frequency. There are thousands, if not hundreds of thousands of other empaths out there who are all devoted to supporting this healing journey that we are collectively going through at this time.

All you are required to do to contribute is learn how to master yourself and contribute in the way that genuinely feels right for you. By learning how to master your own energies, you can put yourself and your purpose to positive use and change the world immediately around you. You can do this by being a local energy healer, teacher, or philosopher if doing something more intimate feels right for you, or you can do this by pursuing a wide-scale mission such as having a public talk show to reach the masses. There is absolutely nothing that states that one dream or purpose is any more or less than another, no matter how large or small either may seem. You must trust that you were born with the divine capacity to fulfill your purpose and that your purpose is exactly what you feel is your calling in life, no matter what anyone says or thinks about it. Some of the most impactful callings of empaths came from innovating a new way by contributing their own energy and purpose into the collective and serving in the way that felt right to them. There is no right or wrong way to contribute.

If you are not yet sure as to what your personal calling is, chances are that you are struggling to spend that time with yourself and gain your self-awareness around it because you are feeling strapped down by the constant energy drainage of society. Do not worry, your calling will appear and show itself to you when the time is right. All you need to do is stay on track, pursue your healing journey, and do what feels right for you. Before you know it, it will appear and you will have the exact blueprint for what you are here to accomplish in life.

Chapter 2: Signs of Being an Empath

If you read through chapter 1 and found yourself feeling a deep resonance with the examples you were reading, you can pretty much already guarantee that you are an empath. However, you may find yourself wondering exactly what your empathic gift entails and what aspects of yourself is a reflection of your gift. Being an empath shows up in many ways, so chances are you have encountered many instances where empathy has impacted or changed your life and how you interact with the world around you.

To help you feel confident that you are an empath, as well as to help you understand exactly how being an empath is impacting your life, we are going to explore the signs of empathy and the common symptoms empaths experience in their lives. This is going to help you determine if you truly are an empath and how your life is being impacted by empathy.

Although many signs are listed in this chapter, you may not experience all of them in your own life. Each empath is slightly unique in the way that their gift manifests. Therefore, you may find yourself deeply resonating with some of these signs more than others. You may also find yourself agreeing with each of them to some degree. As long as you can deeply resonate with at least three or four of these signs, chances are that you are an empath. It is likely that you will be experiencing more or experiencing these signs to a deeper level as you dive further into your gift and embrace the reality of being an empath.

29 Signs of Being an Empath

People Point Out Your Sensitivity

Other people have a tendency to recognize increased sensitivity in empaths, often pointing it out to them during various points in your life. In the past, your increased sensitivity may have been praised as a wonderful sign of you having a big heart, or it may have been used against you in those who claim that your sensitivity is a weakness. Either way, people pointing out your sensitivity is a common experience that empaths encounter in their lives.

Being sensitive to the point of having others recognize that sensitivity may feel either like a blessing or a curse depending on how it has been displayed to you by others. If you have regularly been bullied around your sensitivity, you may feel that this is a weakness and that you have to try and be stronger and have a harder "shell." In this case, you are going to need to heal your inner child from these instances of bullying so that you can embrace your sensitivity as a gift. If you have had it construed as a positive thing in your life, such as people commenting on how much they appreciate you being a sensitive person, you might find yourself sometimes being exploited for your sensitivity. While this is not always the case, many empaths have a tendency to lean into people pleasing and "giving away" their energy through their sensitivity in order to maintain a positive environment around others.

You Feel Other's Feelings

If you are around people and you begin genuinely experiencing the emotions that they themselves are experiencing, you are likely an empath. Empaths often report deeply feeling the emotions of others, often even expressing them more clearly and effectively than the other person might be. For example, if someone comes across bad news and feels a sense of shock and sadness, you might find yourself experiencing the intense energy and even crying from the news despite the fact that it does not impact you. This display may be even more "showy" than the other person who may struggle to effectively feel and process their emotions.

On that note, being around people who do not know how to effectively process their emotions may be extremely overwhelming for you. Around individuals who have a tendency to bottle their emotions up, you might feel a constant, intense feeling inside that comes from having too many unexpressed emotions. Alternatively, around individuals who have a tendency to express themselves loudly or even aggressively, you may also feel overwhelmed because the output of energy is so intense and you feel that energy within yourself.

Negative Feelings Overwhelm You

Empaths often find themselves feeling overwhelmed by negative feelings. This includes the negative feelings of others as well as the negative feelings of themselves. Negative feelings often come with a heavy, dense energy that can leave an empath feeling as though they are being literally weighted down by the emotion itself. As a result, it can lead to exhaustion, frustration, and difficulty expressing yourself. An intense desire to get the energy away from you may lead to you avoiding negative feelings or even denying them as a way to avoid having to face that heavy denseness.

A surprising thing that many empaths do not realize is that positive feelings can become overwhelming, too. Positive energy emits at a high frequency and can lead to feelings that are similar to anxiety, especially if experienced for longer periods of time. It is not unusual for an empath to feel particularly drained after a positive experience because the frequency of energy was rather high and intense.

Crowded Spaces Are Overwhelming

If you are an empath who has not yet healed and mastered your gift, you likely find yourself feeling extremely overwhelmed in crowded areas. Anywhere with a large gathering of people may feel draining because of the sheer amount of energies that you are constantly absorbing and processing. You may feel as though you yourself are moving in slow motion as the energies around you are moving at rabbit speed. The two completely opposite frequencies can lead to an intense sense of overwhelm that can cause anything from exhaustion and a desire to leave early to severe anxiety and a desire to avoid all crowds altogether at any cost.

If you find yourself experiencing intense anxiety around crowds yet you prefer to be an outgoing and extroverted person, the inner conflict may be extremely frustrating as you attempt to balance your anxiety with your extroverted desires. The good thing is, through learning how to master your energy and manage yourself in places with busier energies, you can actually change the way you approach crowds and successfully engage in and even thrive in extroverted experiences.

Your Intuition Is Strong

In a world where everyone seems to be striving to get back in touch with their intuition, you may struggle to relate to this desire. To you, being in touch with your intuition is something that has always come naturally to you and you might find yourself feeling surprised that it is not the same for others. For as long as you can remember, you have always experienced input from your intuition and it has always been right. Whether or not you chose to believe it or follow it, however, may be a completely different story.

Because of how "hard" society has been for so long, many empaths find themselves blatantly ignoring their intuition and following what they were "supposed" to do instead. Often, this result in them being drawn down the wrong path and doing the wrong things which can lead to a myriad of problems and consequences. If you have found yourself struggling to trust your intuition despite it always seeming correct in the end, you are not alone. As you heal your relationship with yourself and your higher consciousness, your ability to trust in and act on your intuition will increase and you will find yourself not struggling nearly as much.

Your Pain Threshold Is Low

Many empaths find that their actual pain threshold for both physical and emotional experiences is particularly low. Getting your vaccine shots, dealing with a paper cut, or even feeling a headache may feel particularly intense for you. You may have even found it to be so bad that you are embarrassed to experience these things around others for fear of how they may react to your response to a painful stimulus.

You might find yourself avoiding places that include a lot of pain, such as doctors' offices or hospitals, because being around so many people who are in pain is challenging for you. To you, not only do the others in pain create a difficult energy for you to embrace, but so does the energy of the building itself. You prefer to avoid these places as often as possible so that you do not have to embrace the energy of pain.

Your Physical Awareness Is Strong

People likely don't believe you about this, but you can feel when you are getting sick before any symptoms even begin arising. You may sense that there is something in your body creating sickness and have the ability to recognize what changes are happening within your body as a result, even if those changes are nothing significant. Sometimes, you may not even be able to describe them as any particular symptom because, for you, it is so subtle yet still so obvious. The same likely goes for headaches, gastrointestinal disorders, and muscle pain.

Some people may consider you to be a hypochondriac because you are constantly reflecting on changes within your body and, in some cases; you may find yourself worried that something bad is happening. When you attempt to explain things to doctors, they may struggle to get a clear diagnosis for you because what you are experiencing is something that most don't speak about so they cannot connect the symptoms to any recognized diseases. It is likely that most people experience these symptoms but fail to recognize them because they lack the keen physical awareness that you have. Regardless, your concerns do have merit and, in the end, there is often a discovery of something that could be causing your symptoms. The primary reason why they were not considered previously is that your doctor likely failed to recognize that you had noticed them sooner than others would have and so, they assumed that the probable causes were unlikely.

You Avoid Negative Media and Images

When you come across media or images that are negative in nature, you may find yourself quickly looking away to avoid the intense energetic response that you have to experience. Seeing images of cruelty or hearing stories of pain that was experienced by others likely makes you feel extremely uncomfortable. You may find yourself feeling nauseated and almost sickened by the stories that you hear or the pictures that you see. You may also feel an intense outburst of pain almost as though the suffering has been caused onto you as well.

It is likely that you have created an environment where you avoid paying attention to the news, reading tabloids, or scrolling certain social media pages because you fear the pain that you will experience if you come across a negative article. Rather than risking it, you would prefer to avoid it and keep your energy feeling safe and free of any feelings of sickness or pain from these types of stories or images.

You Can Spot a Liar

People likely cannot lie around you as you can intuitively tell anytime someone is not telling you the truth. Although you likely cannot explain it, you can feel inside anytime someone tells you or someone around you a lie or purposefully holds back the truth. There is an energy to it that makes you feel skeptical and uncomfortable and that supports you in believing that what they have said is dishonest.

The energy experienced by people who lie may feel extremely uncomfortable for you, so you may find yourself avoiding liars altogether. If someone you know or spend time with is a perpetual liar, you likely minimize your time around them or find a polite way to end your relationship to avoid being in the presence of that energy. The feeling itself is uncomfortable and can be extremely draining, and furthermore, you do not want to spend your time around liars. As such, you avoid these relationships like the plague.

Stimulants or Medications Seem Stronger

When you take a stimulant or medication, or anything else that could in some way "intoxicate" you, you likely find yourself being impacted far greater than the average person. For example, caffeine may have a particularly increased impact on you by causing you to feel excessively energized anytime you ingest it. Drinking alcohol may be something that you have to do in intense moderation to avoid overdoing it, and in some cases, it can even make your empathic gifts more overwhelming than normal.

Many empaths state that they struggle to even take ibuprofen for headaches because they have such a strong impact on them. Because of your increased physical awareness, you may also find yourself struggling to embrace the physical differences that come with taking medications such as painkillers. Any time you feel them in your system, it may create a sense of discomfort or anxiety that lasts until the medication fully leaves your system. This can lead you to avoiding painkillers and leaning towards natural remedies instead, which leave you feeling better in the end.

You Experience Other's Symptoms

A common and sometimes strange symptom that people experience when they are empaths is the ability to experience other people's symptoms. If you have ever been around someone who reported experiencing a certain symptom, such as a headache, and then you began feeling a headache come on yourself, you are an empath. This particular dynamic can feel challenging because others may feel as though you are trying to compete with them and their symptoms as a way to gain attention from others. The reality is, this is not happening at all. What is happening instead is that you feel sympathetic to this person to such an intense degree that you take on their symptom.

A common and sometimes humorous instance where this happens is with sympathetic pregnancies experienced by husbands or other people who are particularly closed to pregnant women. For example, if a husband is in the labor room with his laboring wife and he begins experiencing what feels to be contractions, he is experiencing sympathetic labor. Empaths get this often, and sometimes with people that they do not even necessarily know. Because empaths tend to be sympathetic towards *everyone,* they can pick up these strange symptoms from anyone, sometimes even without having that person actually say anything about the symptom they are experiencing.

You Attract Narcissistic People

One unfortunate side effect of being an empath is that you likely have a tendency to attract narcissistic people into your life. Narcissists are people who completely lack the capacity to experience empathy to any degree whatsoever. While they can effectively mimic signs of empathy, they cannot genuinely feel it in themselves which often results in them frequently engaging in harmful and hurtful behaviors. Narcissists tend to be very abusive and manipulative and are known to cause immense psychological and emotional suffering to their "victims."

As an empath, you have the one thing that narcissists completely lack: empathy. Furthermore, you have an excess of it in comparison to other people. As a result, you are an ideal candidate for them to latch onto because they know that you are more likely to be empathetic towards them and their internal suffering. On some level, you can feel the pain that they experience that has led to them being incapable of having empathy for themselves or anyone around them and this leads to you feeling sorry for them. You may even find yourself trying to fix them, even though they cannot be fixed. In the end, you just end up getting manipulated and hurt by the narcissist and the cycle never truly ends, nor will it. You have to learn to end relationships with narcissists and remove the belief that you are responsible for their ability to heal themselves when they are not willing or capable of truly healing.

If you are engaged in a relationship with a narcissist, you would benefit from reading up on narcissism and understanding what these relationships are like and why they will never change. This can help you end your relationship with narcissists and avoid entering future ones so that you can stop being exploited by people who lack the capacity to genuinely understand that they are exploiting you.

Others Come To You for Support

You have a tendency to be extremely compassionate towards others when they are going through pain because you "get" them in a way that no one else really can. As a result, you likely find a lot of people coming to you for support. You may even find that people you have never met before seem to know that you are supportive and empathetic and so they open up to you without truly knowing who you are. Of course, you support them nonetheless because that is who you are, just as they suspected.

Supporting others seems to be a natural gift of yours, and sometimes, you may find yourself even doing it to the point of your own detriment. Your empathy may make it hard for you to recognize when you need to stop supporting others and offer the support to yourself instead, so you may find yourself giving too much of yourself and your energy to others from time to time.

You Experience Fatigue Often

The constant absorption and expression of energy that you experience within you and around you can lead you to feeling a constant sense of exhaustion. Sometimes, the exhaustion may feel purely mental and you might feel as though your physical body could continue going for quite some time. This type of fatigue may lead to brain fog, difficulty concentrating, and an inability to truly engage in the environment around you. As a result, you find yourself retreating to rest and do nothing, even though physically, you could easily keep going if you wanted to.

This doesn't mean you don't experience physical fatigue too, though. In fact, you may find yourself feeling completely mentally and physically exhausted even after a day of doing almost nothing. Simply sitting at a desk working can seem physically and mentally exhausting to you if you are surrounded by too many people. Even a basic outing like grocery shopping or clothes shopping may overwhelm you and lead to you feeling as though you cannot possibly function without a good rest. While other people do things at all hours of the day, you may find yourself planning your outings around rest periods so that you can slow down and catch up after all of the exhaustion that you experience.

Your Inner Life Is Very Vibrant

Empaths tend to have a very vibrant inner world. You may find yourself rich with visions, dreams, ideas, and hopes that you hold onto and cultivate on a regular basis. If you are left to your own devices, chances are that you find yourself engaging in these inner experiences and spending time daydreaming, creating, or even enjoying more mystical experiences like astral traveling or lucid dreaming.

Unlike others, you find your alone time to be enriching and enjoyable because of the sheer amount of things that you have to think about, dream up, and create. In fact, you may find that if you do not get enough time alone to engage in your inner world, you feel overwhelmed and frustrated. You regularly schedule a time to be alone and enjoy things by yourself and this supports you in feeling enriched and lively so that you can enjoy life in a more vibrant and fulfilling way.

You Experience Sensitivity to Sounds and Sensations

Sounds and sensations have a tendency to create extremely overwhelming energies within you if you are not careful. As an empath, you may find that certain sounds or even the volume of different sounds can lead to you feeling overwhelmed and exhausted. You might also find that certain sounds and sensations can stimulate other sensations within you that create a sense of pain or discomfort. Many people understand what it is like to listen to nails on a chalkboard or the jiggling of keys and feel a shiver up and down their spine. For you, you likely have many triggers that can cause these types of uncomfortable sensations that are not strictly associated with sounds.

You might also find that other sounds or sensations create a particular sensation within you that feels incredibly good. For example, certain relaxing soundtracks may lead to you feeling a genuine sense of calm almost instantly that can easily override any emotion that you were experiencing before. You may find yourself populating your environment with different sounds and textures as well as lights and visual aids that support you in creating these positive and enjoyable sensations.

Multi-Tasking Overwhelms You

Attempting to accomplish too many different things at once may lead to you feeling extremely overwhelmed and exhausted.

Attempting to do something even as simple as eat and watch a movie, for example, can lead to you feeling like too much is happening and can cause you to feel overwhelmed. This gets especially worse when you attempt to combine too many different things, such as completing a task while holding a conversation and trying to jot down notes about something at the same time. Or, if you go grocery shopping and you are trying to keep track of your list while navigating a busy aisle and listening to your spouse, you may get particularly overwhelmed.

Oftentimes, the feelings of overwhelm that you encounter when you are attempting to do too many things at once likely leads to you feeling frustrated and irritated. You may find that when you are multitasking, you are quick to say something unkind or harsh to someone else because you are having a hard time focusing and you feel frustrated. This can lead to feelings of guilt and even further frustration that simply lead to a strong and challenging spiral of negativity from your attempt to multi-task. Because you know multi-tasking can bring so much frustration, you likely attempt to avoid it at all costs.

You Have To Manage Your Environment

It is not unusual for an empath to feel as though they have to manage their own environment. Trying to gain a sense of control over your environment by managing everything and everyone that comes into it is likely your way of making sure that the energies do not become overwhelming. If you are in an environment that you struggle to manage, you might find yourself feeling as though you have to leave the environment because you simply cannot mesh into it effectively.

In your home, it is likely that you are fairly particular not only about how things look but also about how they *feel.* You probably decorate and organize in a way that feels good to you, even if it does not necessarily make sense to anyone else. To others, your environment might look confused or disoriented, but to you, it looks absolutely perfect.

You Don't Enjoy Being Around Selfish People

When you are around anyone who behaves in a selfish way, you likely find yourself immediately trying to leave the vicinity and end your engagements with them. People who are selfish have a tendency to bring up feelings of frustration and anxiety in empaths because they can become energetic vampires who suck up your energy. This can feel draining, overwhelming, and downright exhausting.

If you are in a relationship with someone who is selfish and you cannot end it, such as a relationship with a selfish boss or sibling, you might find yourself trying to create as much distance in that relationship as possible. By avoiding them, minimizing the time you spend communicating, and trying to buffer your encounters with another person, you feel as though you can avoid being drained by this person.

You Can Feel Things That Don't Have Feelings

Others might say it is strange, but you can literally feel the energy of the things that are around you. Things that do not even have feelings, like inanimate objects or even days of the week may possess a very real and very strong energy in your mind. For example, if you see a toy on the wrong shelf and a group of the same toys all on a different shelf, you may feel compelled to return the oddly placed object to its group. To you, it may feel sad or lonely so you need to put it back with the rest of its "friends."

Things like days of the week, seasons, and even just specific words all have the energy to you, too. If you were to wake up on a Sunday, for example, it would have a completely different energy than a Tuesday just based off of the day itself and without any regard to the contents of your calendar or the mood of anyone around you. You may also feel a certain sense of joy around specific positive words and a sense of nagging suffering around specific negative words. These energies may not make sense to anyone but you, but you are certain that you can feel them and they impact you in a big way.

Listening is One of your Strengths

In any conversation, you are a great listener. You can intuitively "hear" everything the person is not saying over the top of what they are saying which leads to you having the capacity to somehow know what they mean or feel even if they have struggled to effectively communicate themselves. This ability to hear the unspoken information means that you can understand people in a way that others don't. People often feel very well-received around you and as though they can express themselves in a more authentic way because they know that you will "get it."

You may even find yourself actively engaged in a career or hobbies that revolve around you listening because you are so good at it. To you, it may feel good or even fascinating to be able to listen to people and hear everything they are and are not saying and provide them with a sense of true understanding. This is especially true if you have the empathic calling of the healer or the teacher.

Boredom Tends To Creep In Often

Your rich inner world and your constant energetic alertness can create incredibly wonderful and enriching experiences in your life. However, it can also result in you feeling extremely bored and withdrawn in certain circumstances, too. Trying to engage in mundane tasks like listening to board meetings or inputting data into computers can feel extremely boring to you because your mind wants to be actively engaged and working. It is used to being "on the go," and so, anytime you are stationary or have slowed down, it grows frustrated and tries to find new things to do.

As a way to curb your boredom, you may find yourself regularly leaning towards engaging in more enriching experiences that draw out your natural talents for communication or creation. These types of experiences allow you to play with energy in a more enjoyable manner and support you in feeling better in your life. When you engage in these experiences, you can feel your energy coming out to play and the experience likely fulfills your entire sense of being with feelings of joy and satisfaction.

You Might Be Introverted

Many empaths find themselves experiencing an introverted lifestyle because they struggle to engage in active or overwhelming environments. To empaths who are naturally introverted or who are inexperienced with managing their energy in a healthier way, isolating themselves may be an opportunity to cut themselves off from the overly energetic outside world. By retreating into an introverted lifestyle, empaths can minimize the amount of energy around them and feel more confident in controlling themselves and their responses to it.

Even empaths who desire to be extroverted likely find themselves retreating as a way to save themselves from the outside energies of the world. This can lead to feelings of inner conflict and frustration as the empath struggles to decide between going out and engaging in the world and feeling overwhelmed or staying home and taking care of their energies.

Intimate Relationships May Feel Overwhelming

For some empaths, being engaged in intimate relationships can be particularly overwhelming. The intimate relationship can feel like an energy pit where the empath is constantly required to invest more of themselves than they comfortably can, even if the relationship follows a healthy dynamic. For an empath who is used to living on their own or being by themselves, welcoming someone new into their space in such a big way can feel overwhelming and frustrating. They may find themselves avoiding intimate relationships altogether so that they can keep a greater control over their personal space.

If you feel like intimate relationships are particularly challenging for you, chances are you are experiencing a common setback for empaths who are not yet clear on how to establish and maintain healthy energetic boundaries between themselves and others. As you learn how to heal your energies and assert your energetic boundaries, building and nurturing intimate relationships will begin to feel a lot easier for you.

Nature Feels Nourishing To You

Empaths often have incredible experiences in nature. While nature itself is beautiful for anyone who chooses to enjoy time in it, empaths find themselves literally needing to get into nature as a way to nurture their sense of wellbeing and release the energy build-ups they may be experiencing. Nature is a grounding space for empaths to go to that supports them in finally feeling free to just *be.*

If you find that nature itself is like a friend to you that supports you in living your best life, it is likely because nature is where you gain the opportunity to finally feel at peace in your life. Spending plenty of time in nature can support you in feeling nurtured and healed so that you can continue enjoying your life to the fullest. You can also bring nature indoors with house plants and pets who can support you in feeling connected to the beauty of nature without having to spend all of your time outside.

You Have a Big Heart

You are likely an extremely loving and kindhearted person. Empaths are known for their big hearts and their ability to show love to many different people without reserve or inhibition. Empaths rarely feel as though love needs to be "earned" or given in any form of slow distribution. They are happy to share their love and kindness with anyone who they may cross paths with and they do it from the generosity of their own heart. Empaths do not distribute great amounts of love because they expect to be loved back, but they do so because the energy of love is genuinely fulfilling to an empath and they love sharing it with everyone.

If you find yourself dropping bits of love here and there and the heart emoji is one of your most used emojis, chances are you are an empath. Your desire to spread love everywhere to everyone comes from your inner divine purpose of healing the collective through love and compassion. The more you engage in sharing the love with those around you, the better you are going to feel overall.

Your Search for Truth

Empaths strongly dislike the energy associated with lies and dishonesty so they often find themselves searching for the truth in life. They like to surround themselves with honest people who are also in pursuit of the truth as their energy tends to feel more "pure" and "clean." Empaths can easily detect the dishonesty in the media, politics, and even in education that is taught to them. They rarely allow themselves to fall into the traps of society and are almost always looking for ways to embody and embrace collective truth and their personal truth into their own life.

If you find yourself skeptical over what the collective tends to see as "true" and you are regularly searching for ways to understand what the real truth is, chances are you are an empath who is in pursuit of honesty. Through finding honesty, empaths are able to support society through healing, teaching, and advocating for the truth and bringing an end to many of the different sufferings society has faced. Thanks to empaths, we are constantly moving toward a new, healthier society.

You Experience Frequent Mood Swings

As an empath who is not actively aware of how they can manage their own energy field in any different situation, you may find yourself experiencing frequent mood swings. Mood swings arise as a result of having your energy tapped out by the people who surround you. This is just like experiencing other people's symptoms, except you also experience their emotions.

In larger crowds or in environments that are particularly emotional, you may find that this symptom is increased. This is because there are far more people with emotions that are surrounding you and impacting your energy. However, it can still happen in quiet and calm environments. Even the simple energy change of weather, the hour on the clock, or the energy of your environment (or social media newsfeed) can impact your energy which then impacts your mood.

Beating around the Bush is not your Thing

One symptom many empaths experience is their bluntness. Beating around the bush is not common with empaths. They realize that holding back the truth or trying to say it in a nicer way can defeat the purpose of the message and prevent the other person from fully understanding. Even if it is hard and uncomfortable, an empath will almost always tell it like it is.

Chapter 3: The Empath Phenomenon

The empath phenomenon is a way that psychologists and psychiatrists have managed to look into the world of empathic gifts and discover why empaths feel, think, and act the way that they do. Through looking into the mind of empaths, researchers have discovered five reasons why empaths are this way. What they discovered was how the mirror neuron system, electromagnetic fields, emotional contagion, increased dopamine sensitivity, and synesthesia all come together to support an empath with their gifts.

That's right, there is literally a science behind your gifts that explains why they work the way they do and how they impact you. In this chapter, we are going to explore these five factors and discover how they support you in being an empath. This is going to help you feel more confident in your gift by realizing that it is very normal and that many people experience it. Through understanding the science of empathy, we are also able to discover how healing can take place so that you can heal yourself and experience life as an empowered empath who thrives on a day-to-day basis. This way, you do not have to feel as though you are suffering at the hand of your sensitivity.

The Mirror Neuron System

In your brain, a specific group of specialized brain cells exists solely for the purpose of experiencing compassion. These brain cells work in a way that allows individuals to mirror the emotions or feelings of another individual, such as fear or joy. With these brain cells, we are able to experience compassion for each other so that we can support one another in many different ways throughout life. For example, if your child were crying, you would also feel sad from your mirror neuron system. If your friend was feeling joyful about their recent promotion at work, you would feel joy with them, too. Through this ability to mirror another's emotions, you are able to genuinely share their experience and offer your support in whatever way it may be needed. This helps us deepen our emotional connections and supports us in experiencing a stronger sense of community with those around us.

Empaths are believed to have a set of mirror neuron cells that are hyper-responsive, allowing empaths to resonate at an even deeper level with those around them. This allows empaths to feel even deeper connections with those around them, allowing them to feel as though they can literally feel the emotions or pain of another individual. Because the resonance is deeper and the mirroring is stronger, empaths may even find themselves crying alongside someone who is in pain because they are able to mirror the other person's emotions to such a strong degree.

In contrast to empaths are narcissists, sociopaths, and psychopaths. These are individuals who are believed to have what is known as an "empathy deficient disorder" meaning that their mirror neuron system is actually underactive. These individuals are incapable of experiencing unconditional love and have a tendency to cause harm to others as a way to feel good in their own life. They are known to cling to empaths or individuals who experience higher levels of empathy likely because they long to feel empathy themselves but cannot produce empathetic emotions on their own.

Electromagnetic Fields

Science has shown that the heart and the brain are both actively capable of producing electromagnetic fields that are pulsated into the space around the individual. The HeartMath Institute claims that these electromagnetic fields have the capacity to transmit information about a person's energy, such as their emotions (energy in motion,) to other people. In general, everyone can intuitively sense and pick up information from these electromagnetic fields even if they do not realize that they are actively doing it. However, it is believed that empaths are more sensitive to these energy fields and that they can become overwhelmed by it often because they do not know what is happening and they may not be able to tell the difference between their own electromagnetic field and someone else's.

Other individuals are not the only ones equipped with electromagnetic fields, either. The moon, the sun, the earth, and many other things exist with their own electromagnetic fields that we can intuitively pick up. Just like with other humans, empaths are believed to be more in tune with these electromagnetic fields, too. Most empaths believe without a fraction of a doubt that the sun, moon, and earth can significantly impact their energy and mind from the electromagnetic output. That being said, not all realize that it is from the science-backed electromagnetic field that exists around various people and things.

Emotional Contagion

A phenomena known as "emotional contagion" is believed to be a part of an empaths ability to feel other people to such a strong degree, too. Research has shown that the average individual can sense and pick up on the emotions of others when they are nearby. Emotional contagion can best be recognized in a household where one person comes home grumpy after a bad day and then everyone else seems to find themselves feeling grumpy, too. People can generally "catch" someone else's feelings and they can spread like a wave over a group of people, quickly bringing many individuals into the same emotional experience.

Psychologists believe that emotional contagion is how groups of people are able to maintain great relationships: because they are able to intimately understand each other and express similar emotions and understanding. As you may have expected, it is believed that empaths have a stronger capacity to "catch" other people's feelings through this very phenomena. As such, they find themselves feeling other people's emotions in a particularly intense manner that may feel as though the emotion is authentically their own when, in reality, it came from someone else.

Increased Dopamine Sensitivity

Dopamine is a neurotransmitter that is known for increasing the activity of neurons in the brain. Dopamine is associated with responses including pleasure. Research was done that suggested that empaths who identify as introverts are known for having a higher sensitivity to dopamine than extroverts have. What this means is that an introverted empath requires less dopamine in order to feel a pleasurable response to stimuli in their environment. This likely explains why introverted empaths are more content doing something quiet and relaxed than something outgoing: too much stimulation that produces too much dopamine could result in feelings of overwhelm and anxiety from significantly increased pleasure.

Empaths who identify as extroverted are still particularly sensitive to dopamine, but it was recognized that the way they process dopamine is fairly different from introverted empaths.

Rather than feeling overwhelmed by an excess of it, extroverted empaths actually crave dopamine and find themselves doing things in search of an "increased dopamine high." This means that they will regularly engage in active environments, join crowds, and enjoy the more outgoing side of life as a way to feel fueled up and positive in their life.

Synesthesia

There is a state known as "mirror-touch synesthesia" which seems to be the most aligned with the empath phenomenon. Synesthesia itself is a neurological condition that is known for pairing two completely different senses together in the brain. For example, if you hear a certain piece of music and you begin seeing certain colors in your mind's eye, you are experiencing synesthesia.

Mirror-touch synesthesia is an amplified variation of this condition whereby individuals can actually feel the emotions and sensations of other people within their own body. The way they feel these sensations seem as though they are actually happening to them when, in reality, they are not. However, an empath would likely not know the difference since they may have no idea what is actually going on. To them, it may feel so compelling that they genuinely believe their emotions are being impacted by something happening directly to them. Not only does this phenomenon clearly explain what happens to empaths during their empathic experiences, but it also gives a very clear reason as to why these things are happening.

As you now realize, being an empath is a very real experience and it is largely involved in electromagnetic fields and mirror-touch synesthesia. The question now is: how can you incorporate healing into your life so that you can gain more control over these experiences and stop feeling as though you are entrapped in a vicious cycle that you cannot escape? The answer is somewhat simple: you need to begin engaging in healing. One way that you can begin healing is through energy healing which is designed to support you in keeping your own electromagnetic fields clear and comfortable. You also need to focus on living life for yourself and taking back any control that you may have lost through previous traumatic or painful experiences. By healing from your past and allowing yourself to take back control, you can take control over your energies and begin living your best life.

Chapter 4: Energetic Healing Practices

Energetic healing practices are one of the most important healing practices that an empath can begin learning about. Energetic healing practices enable empaths to begin the healing process right away without having to engage in past, present or future psychological healing. While these types of psychological healings are still beneficial, and in many cases necessary, you can begin experiencing a significant amount of relief from your symptoms just by engaging in energetic healing practices.

When it comes to energetic healing practices, there are two ways that you can choose to go that will provide you with great support and benefits. One includes having a trained practitioner conduct your healing for you and the other includes you conducting the healing on yourself. Ideally, you should be engaging in both styles in order to gain maximum healing benefits. During times where you want to practice extra self-care or experience an approach that is more hands-off for you, going to an energy healer who is trained in any modality that feels fitting for you is effective. For periods in between your sessions, knowing how to heal your own energy empowers you to stay in control over your energy and maintain an optimal state of energetic health.

In this chapter, we are going to explore the many varieties of energy healing available and how you can utilize them in your own life. Many of these energy healing practices can be done on your own *or* with the experienced support of a practitioner so that you can gain full benefits of your energy healing experience. If you have never experienced energy healing before, you can still engage in these practices to begin taking back control over your energy right now!

Acupuncture

Acupuncture is a type of energy healing that must be done by experienced practitioners as it is completed in a very specific manner. With acupuncture, small needles are inserted into your skin at various meridians around the body. Meridians are areas where energy is believed to build up and sometimes become "stuck" within the body. By gently tapping the needles into these meridians, it is believed that balance can be restored within the body.

This modality of healing stems from ancient Chinese medicine practices where it was designed to support individuals in releasing chronic pain, as well as emotional and spiritual pain. This energy modality works with the psychosomatic system to support complete energetic healing in anyone who experiences it. You can have acupuncture done by a professionally trained therapist who is capable of considering your energetic healing needs and promoting energy flow within your body using acupuncture.

Chakra Clearing

Chakra is a Sanskrit word for "wheel" or "disk" which is used to reference seven energy centers that are positioned throughout the human body. These energy centers are located at the base of your spine, slightly below your belly button, in your solar plexus, over your heart, in your throat, slightly above and between your eyebrows, and at the crown of your head. Each one is assigned its own color, name, and meaning for what it represents within your body, life, and spiritual self.

Empaths who are not actively clearing their energy on a regular basis have a tendency to find their chakras either overactive or underactive. In either state, the chakra is believed to produce an unhealthy balance within the individual that can lead to negative or unwanted energetic experiences. For example, an overactive third eye chakra (the one located slightly above and between your eyebrows) can result in you experiencing excessive visions or mental stimulation. An underactive third eye chakra can result in you struggling to experience any vision at all, maybe even finding yourself incapable of using your imagination or engaging in creative thought.

Knowing how to clear your chakras starts with being able to locate them and sense them. A great way to do this is to lie on your back, allow yourself to relax into a meditative state, and then hover your hand about six inches over your body. Start by hovering it over top of your root chakra and see if you can sense any energy coming from it. Then, move your hand up your body as you "read" each of your seven chakras. Getting a feel for what your chakras feel like in this way is a wonderful opportunity to start exploring and understanding your chakras and how they feel to you.

Once you have located your chakras, you can begin practicing chakra clearing with each of your chakras. Typically, each chakra requires its own unique balancing practice unless you are using Reiki which addresses each chakra in one healing. You can balance each chakra based on which ones you feel are overactive or underactive from your body scan.

I have listed each chakra's name, color, meaning, and healing practice below.

- **Root Chakra** (*Muladhara*) located at the base of your spine. This chakra is red in color and represents your connection to Earth and the lower portion of your body (i.e. legs, knees, and feet). You can heal your root chakra by walking barefoot in nature, by spending time in nature, or by eating healthy red foods like tomatoes, berries, and apples.

- **Sacral Chakra** (*Swadhisthana)* located slightly below your belly button. This chakra is orange in color and represents your creativity and your reproductive organs. You can heal your sacral chakra by swimming or spending time in a relaxing bath, or by eating orange foods like carrots, melons, mangoes, or oranges.

- **Solar Plexus Chakra** (*Manipura*) located over your solar plexus. This chakra is yellow in color and represents your personal power and connection to your true essence. The solar plexus chakra affects your digestive system. You can heal your solar plexus chakra by spending time in the bright sun, by enjoying a nice fire or by eating yellow foods like bananas, pineapple, turmeric or corn.
- **Heart Chakra** (*Anahata*) located over your heart. This chakra is green in color and represents your emotions. It affects your heart system and all organs associated with blood flow. You can heal your heart chakra by breathing in fresh air or spending time with your windows open. You can also heal it by eating foods that are rich with chlorophyll like avocado, broccoli, and all leafy greens.

- **Throat Chakra** (*Vishuddha*) located in your throat. This chakra is blue in color and represents your ability to speak kindly and clearly to others. It affects your throat, your mouth, and oral health. You can heal your throat chakra by singing, sitting under a bright blue sky or eating blue foods like blueberries, dragon fruit, or currants.

- **Third Eye Chakra** (*Ajna*) located between and slightly above your eyebrows. This chakra is indigo and represents your ability to experience visions, imaginative thinking, and "see" into the spiritual world. It affects your brain and eyes. You can clear your third eye chakra by sitting in the sunlight or by eating indigo foods like grapes and blackberries.

- **Crown Chakra** (*Sahasrara*) located at the crown of your head and slightly above your head. This chakra is violet and represents your ability to stay connected to Source. It also affects your brain as well as your energy body and aura. You can heal your crown chakra by connecting with all of the elements including earth, water, air, and fire. The crown chakra is heavily connected to spirit so it is not associated with any particular food sources.

Crystal Healing

Crystals are a wonderful way to support yourself in experiencing a healing, nourished energy body. You can use crystal healing during specific sessions such as in meditation, or you can use crystal healing by carrying a crystal with you as you go about your daily activities. Crystals and gemstones have the capacity to support your body, mind, and spirit in feeling their very best when it comes to energy. You can use crystals as a way to draw impurities out of your energy body, to balance energies within the body or even to inspire and promote certain energies in your body.

When it comes to an official healing ritual, crystals are often used alongside meditation by being placed upon the body in what is known as a "crystal grid." This is done by laying crystals over your body at certain points depending on where the energy is most needed. There are many different crystal varieties available to individuals, so the best way to ensure that you are using the proper crystals is to consider what your energy needs are (i.e. more loving energy) and pick the appropriate crystal for such healing purpose (i.e. rose quartz). Then, you can lay your crystals over the areas of your body where you would like to send or remove that particular energy from the body. For example, if you wanted to protect your third eye, you could place a piece of amethyst over your third eye.

If you are looking to get a complete crystal healing done, getting one done with a crystal healing practitioner is the best way to make sure that the proper crystals are being laid over the proper areas to promote your healing. Your practitioner may also be able to support you in finding ways that you can use crystal healing at home so that you can practice it on yourself, too.

When it comes to wearing crystals as an opportunity to receive healing from them, there are nearly endless ways that this can be accomplished. Crystals can be worn as earrings, necklaces, bracelets, and even as hair clips or accessories for your clothes. Some people will also use pocket crystals, which are small flat tumbled stones that can be carried in your pocket and, if you feel like it, you can rub them between your fingers throughout the day.

Choosing the right crystals for your healing practices ultimately depends on what you are looking for in your healing. There are crystals for virtually every purpose, so the best way to determine which ones you need is to attend a metaphysical store and request the individual working at the store to support you in finding the right crystals. If you are looking for crystals specifically associated with healing for empaths, there are seven great stones for you to consider including in your collection.

These seven stones include:

- **Black Tourmaline** which is an excellent stone for protecting your energies and preventing unwanted energies from entering your auric body. Any energy that is attempting to have a negative impact on you will be pushed away by the energy of the black tourmaline if you keep a piece on or with you. Black tourmaline is best worn as a pendant or kept in your pocket.

- **Lepidolite** is a great healing stone when it comes to anxiety experienced by empaths. Using lepidolite, you can lessen the anxiety around the energies you are sensing and experiencing so that you can approach life more intentionally and with a calmer energy. The best way to use lepidolite is to meditate with it over your heart chakra or your third eye chakra or to wear it as a pendant.

- **Black Obsidian** is another great stone for protecting you from unwanted energies. Carrying a piece with you or keeping it in your surrounding space is a great way to gain the benefits of black obsidian. It can be quite sharp so it is best to avoid wearing this stone or carrying it in your pocket. You can also meditate with it near your root chakra if you want to use it during a meditation practice.

- **Malachite** is an incredible stone for dealing with emotions and releasing emotional and energetic blockages from your energy body. Malachite is excellent for anyone who encounters stressful situations on a regular basis and who needs to be protected from those stressors. Malachite is best worn as a pendant or meditated with as it rests over your heart chakra.

- **Hematite** is well-known for having many healing benefits to those who wear it. For empaths, hematite is a great stone for supporting you in staying grounded and avoiding harmful energies that may attempt to access your energy body. You can use hematite to avoid people who may try to suck up your energy, such as energy vampires. Hematite is best kept in your pocket or placed near your root chakra when you meditate.

- **Amethyst** is an incredible crystal that is known for its spiritually protective properties. When used in healing, amethyst can protect you from feeling overwhelmed by energies that may be in your immediate surrounding area. It can also be used to help bring a sense of calmness when you enter busier environments or ones that may have stronger or more challenging energies to deal with. Amethyst is excellent for helping empaths decide which energies are theirs and which belong to someone else. You can use amethyst over your third eye in meditation, or worn as nearly any form of jewelry when you go out.

EFT

EFT or Emotional Freedom Techniques® is an energetic healing practice that individuals can practice on themselves after being shown how by an EFT practitioner. The entire practice is based on tapping specific energetic meridians on your body and repeating positive affirmations as you do. The idea is that you are tapping energy lose while replacing it with more positive energy that actually supports you in living a positive and productive life.

Once you have learned how, EFT can easily be practiced by yourself at any given time. However, there are specific meridians and tapping patterns that you need to use in order to gain maximum value from EFT. For that reason, having someone support you in learning how to do it for yourself is the best way to learn how you can use EFT to your healing advantage.

Reiki

Reiki was originally founded by a gentleman named Mikao Usui. The name "Reiki" translates to "spiritually guided life force energy." When individuals engage in Reiki healings, their practitioner channels universal life energy into them as a way to integrate the mind, body, and spirit and encourage natural healing to take place. Thus, the Reiki practitioner is not actually responsible for healing but instead, encourages the universe to produce healing benefits in that specific person.

When Reiki is practiced, it is practiced by someone who has been attuned to Reiki energy by a Reiki instructor. This attunement is considered a necessary initiation to align the practitioner with Spirit energy so that they can begin their journey of energetically healing others. Reiki can be practiced by an attuned practitioner on themselves or on any other consenting individual. This means that if you wanted to, you could become attuned in Reiki healing as a way to begin healing yourself through the magic of Reiki energy.

If you would rather not get attuned in Reiki healing, you can still receive healings from Reiki practitioners. Many of these practitioners will conduct Reiki either face-to-face or through distant sessions which can be completed from virtually anywhere in the world. The reason for this is that Reiki practitioners only need to be able to tune into your energy to direct universal healing energy toward your energy. Since the true healing is coming from Spirit, you are only required to be connected to a source which is an innate gift that you were born with.

Quantum Healing

Quantum healing is similar to Reiki in that it uses life force energy as a way to conduct the healing practice and support healing within the mind, body, and spirit of the receiving individual. While other healings tend to be based on spiritual knowingness and trust, quantum healing is backed by the science of quantum mechanics. This healing modality considers how quantum energy affects the body and how you can focus, amplify, and direct the energy to promote certain healing benefits.

Those who have received quantum healings claim that there are many incredible results from physical to mental and spiritual healing benefits. Often, quantum healing includes a specific breathing practice that supports life force energy in accessing the body and encouraging greater healing experiences.

Qigong

Qigong translates to "vital life force effort." Like Reiki and quantum healing, it also works alongside life force energy as a way to promote energetic healing within the physical body. However, Qigong works through both breathing techniques and meditational practices as a way to stimulate the healing practice and encourage energetic healing within the body. Qigong is a self-healing modality that is taught by individuals trained in Qigong and then practiced by personally by you. You do not have to be trained in Qigong to practice, though it is a good idea to have a trained practitioner to show you how to facilitate the self-healing to ensure that you are using the modality properly.

Qigong practitioners sometimes practice what is known as "Qi emission" which is a style of Qigong that is intended to support the practitioner in directing healing into your body. It is believed that these practices are just as effective, though it does require you to be around a practitioner to gain access to these healing practices. If you want to be able to use Qigong as an energetic healing modality to support you in thriving in life as an empath, learning how to engage in the self-healing modality is the best way to ensure that you are getting maximum benefit from Qigong.

Yoga

Yoga is a physical exercise practice that actually has deep spiritual roots. Yoga is a practice that is used to engage the physical body in various positions that are meant to stimulate energy flow and support individuals in healing whatever may ail them on an energetic or physical level. When you engage in yoga on a regular basis, you ensure that you are allowing energy to successfully flow through you as you also gain the meditational benefits that promote life force energy flow.

You are likely already familiar with yoga and how accessible this healing modality is to people. You can easily engage in yoga by taking part in a local class, or by following one of the many videos available to you in the online space. By engaging in a regular yoga practice, you allow yourself to keep your energy body clear and maintain a more peaceful control over the energy that flows into and out of your auric body.

There are many different styles of yoga, so you may benefit from spending time studying each type of yoga and considering which one may be most beneficial for you based on your unique energetic requirements. You can certainly mix up styles if you desire, but most styles are designed with a specific teaching style in mind. That is, the energetic practices and meditative experiences taught in each style of yoga will vary depending on where it comes from. You will likely find overlapping information in each style, but the way in which it is taught and the methods used to achieve desired outcomes varies between different styles of yoga.

The eleven primary styles of yoga include:

- Hatha yoga
- Iyengar yoga
- Kundalini yoga
- Ashtanga yoga
- Vinyasa yoga
- Bikram yoga
- Yin yoga
- Restorative yoga
- Prenatal yoga
- Anusara yoga
- Jivamukti yoga

The yoga styles that are typically considered best for healing empaths include Hatha yoga, Kundalini yoga, Vinyasa yoga, Yin yoga, Restorative yoga, and Anusara yoga. Each of these styles focuses on spiritual healing in a way that is understandable and accessible for aspiring yogis who are just starting out. None of these practices are necessarily physically demanding nor will they require you to position yourself in any way that may be challenging for someone who is new to yoga. This makes them easy to begin with and extremely supportive when it comes to maintaining your energy balance and feeling confident in your path as an empath.

Chapter 5: Learning To Control Your Energy

A large part of healing your energy is to know how to control your energy in the first place. As an empath, learning how to control your energy gives you the capacity to have a greater say in what comes into your energy field and how it affects you. This is your opportunity to overcome the feelings of being helpless and at the mercy of other energies so that you can feel a greater sense of control and empowerment in your life.

In addition to supporting you in feeling a greater sense of empowerment, learning to control your energies will support you in quickly recognizing when something is off in your energy body. This way, the moment your energies begin to feel overwhelmed, you can prevent them from building up and causing problems by scheduling an energy healing session for yourself.

Controlling your energies ultimately requires three steps: identifying your energies, identifying other people's energies, and setting energetic boundaries so that no one else can interrupt your energy field. In this chapter, we are going to explore how you can begin doing this in your life so that you can gain personal control and feel a greater sense of confidence when going out into the world around you.

Identifying Your Personal Energy

One of the biggest reasons why empaths find themselves feeling vulnerable and overwhelmed is because they struggle to recognize their own energies apart from the energies of others. As a result, they end up feeling as though everything is truly originating from within them and they derive a great sense of overwhelm from struggling to identify why or how it is happening. Once an empath recognizes that many of these energies are not their own, a great sense of relief may be experienced. That great sense of relief may then be followed by a sense of frustration for lacking the knowledge around how to prevent the energy from building up and burdening their energy field.

If you have ever felt yourself feeling frustrated and overwhelmed by other's energies, chances are that you have not yet learned to discern the difference between your own energies and someone else's. That is the first step to learning how to control your energies so that you can refrain from being "hijacked" by someone else's energetic experience and feeling caught at the mercy of those around you. As you learn how to identify your own energies, identifying the energy of other's around you becomes simpler, too. This can take some time and practice, but the more you engage in this practice, the easier it will be for you to recognize your energies versus anyone else's.

The best way to begin is to start by identifying your own energies. When you have a stronger sense of who you are and what your personal energy feels like, it becomes easier for you to identify what energies do not belong to you. Naturally, your own energy field is going to change in accordance with your moods and experiences, so your energy field may not always feel the same. For that reason, you should invest at least several days into the process of getting to know your own personal energy so that you can have a strong sense of what your energy feels like under different circumstances.

Identifying your own energy is as simple as slowing down and tuning in to your inner self. Spending some time in meditation identifying what energy resonates with you the most is a great way to identify your energies. Most people report feeling their personal energy somewhere around their solar plexus chakra, or the core of their physical being. This is believed to be where our personal power comes from, so it makes sense that many people feel their personal energy here. You may feel yours differently, however, so make sure to tune in and consider what genuinely resonates with you. A great way to tell if it is truly your energy is to consider the feeling you get when you hear someone say your name. Typically, this will cause a sensation in your body that result in you perking up and listening to hear who is talking to you. That same familiar sensation is the type you will feel when you have successfully identified your personal energy.

It is a good idea to do small meditative check-ins during the day, too, whenever you experience a variety of different emotions or energies. This allows you to get a sense of what your energy body feels like when you are experiencing different things like anger, fear, joy, gratitude, or even just an excess of energy.

At first, you may find that it is a challenge for you to discover which energies are familiar or feel like yours because you may have spent so much time separated from yourself in this sense. As you continue checking in and recognizing what your own energy feels like that sense of familiarity will continue to rise for you and strengthen your ability to identify your own energies. This way, you can build confidence in yourself and your energy body while also telling yourself apart from others. For an empath, this process alone is a massive step in the right direction.

Identifying Other People's Energies

Once you have successfully identified your own energies, you need to begin identifying what it feels like when someone else's energy penetrates your energy body. When you learn how to identify other people's energies, it becomes even easier for you to draw the barrier between yourself and others in a way that allows you to recognize their energy as their own and your energy as your own.

You have likely already been recognizing other people's energies to some degree even if you do not completely realize it. For example, I bet you can think of one person that makes you feel "off" the minute they enter the room. Perhaps their energy is quite toxic so anytime they are around you; it is as though you can immediately feel the energy in your own space change. You may even find yourself feeling an increased state of fearfulness or overwhelm, likely reflecting the inner pain being experienced by the individual with toxic behaviors. Likewise, you can probably think of someone who has a beautiful energy and who always makes you feel so comforted and welcomed into their space. Maybe you find yourself even craving their presence because it helps you feel so relaxed and at ease in your own life.

Even though not everyone's energy is going to produce such an obvious and profound impact, you are going to be able to experience everyone's energy whether you intend to or not. That is until you begin taking control over your own energy. Learning how to recognize the difference between your energy and someone else's will ensure that you can easily establish that boundary and maintain empathy without physically, mentally, emotionally, or spiritually taking on the other person's experience as though it is your own. The first step is to know how to identify your own energy as this supports you in immediately recognizing what is your own. Then, you need to go ahead and begin identifying everything that is *not* yours as this will clearly tell you which energies you are feeling that belong to someone else.

The best time to practice this is anytime you are in a public setting where you begin to feel overwhelmed. Often, these are the types of environments where the barriers between your energy and other people's energies can blur because you have not yet established healthy energetic boundaries. When you begin feeling this sensation of overwhelm, you need to take action by identifying where the overwhelm is coming from. You can do this through the same self-awareness check-ins that you were using to identify your own energy. First, you need to identify your own energy and develop a sense of familiarity which is going to help ground you and keep you feeling strong in your own space. Then, you need to identify everything that is not your own energy as this is obviously going to be energy that belongs to someone else's. Spend a few minutes visualizing the barrier between your energy and other people's energy so that you can feel confident that there is a difference between the two. This is going to support you in feeling a stronger sense of self which will give you the courage and confidence that you need to take control of your own energy field.

Once you have identified the barrier between yourself and other people, you can take action in two ways. First, you can take action by requesting that any energy that is not inherently yours be removed from your energy field so that you can resume your own natural energetic state. This is going to ensure that any energies that have penetrated your boundaries are removed from your field to promote a feeling of confidence and calm in your own energy. The second thing that you need to do is begin establishing energetic boundaries. These energetic boundaries are going to ensure that your energy field is not regularly being penetrated by the energy of other people. This does not mean that you won't sense and recognize their energy, but it does mean that it will not be able to create a sensation of you being attacked by the energy of others.

The Creation of Energy Boundaries

Creating energy boundaries is a healthy and empowering way of protecting yourself from other people's energies without completely closing yourself off from those around you. When you use energy boundaries, you ensure that the energetic exchange between yourself and someone else does not exceed what feels comfortable and reasonable for you. For example, if you are in the presence of someone who has a toxic energy, your energetic boundary would insist that their toxic energies do not penetrate your energy field. As a result, their toxic energies would still be available for you to see but they would not feel as though they were personally attacking you or entering your sacred personal space. This can support you in overcoming the experience of taking on other people's energies and emotions as though they are your own.

You can create energy boundaries in the same way that you create physical or personal boundaries. Begin by identifying where the boundary is and what it needs to be. For example, if you are feeling overwhelmed by negative energy, then you can set the boundary that other people's negative energy is no longer allowed to become your negative energy. Setting the boundary is as simple as declaring it and becoming conscious of said boundary, the harder part will be your need to assert that boundary and uphold it no matter what.

Upholding the boundary and asserting it as needed requires you to assert it to others either verbally or energetically, as well as uphold it with yourself, too. When it comes to other people bringing negative energy into your space, you can approach the situation in the way that you feel is going to be most effective. If the person is behaving in a way that is toxic, addressing the situation and verbalizing your boundary may be most effective. If they are unaware of their toxicity or they seem to behave in a fairly kind manner but their energy continues to feel toxic, asserting a boundary on an energetic level may be more appropriate. What this means is that you assert to yourself and to your energetic field that no toxic energies will be accepted into your space and then you uphold that assertion by not allowing their energy to impact you any further.

Holding yourself up to boundaries is essential, too. Many people think that the only boundaries that need to be established are the ones that exist between themselves and other people but this is not the case. If you set a boundary and yourself, breach it either towards yourself or towards other people. You are asserting to yourself that this boundary does not matter and that energy can freely leak through it as you will not prevent it from happening. This means that if you assert that you do not want toxic energy in your space, you cannot become toxic towards other people or towards yourself. You need to work towards setting the boundary and eliminating all toxic behaviors, thoughts, and words from your life when you are interacting with yourself or with anyone else. That way, your boundaries are maintained in a healthy way and you can continue growing forward.

Why You Need To Quit Shielding Yourself

Many resources for empaths advocate on the benefits of shielding yourself, and to a degree, they are right. However, maintaining a constant shield over yourself is both ineffective and counterintuitive to what you are attempting to achieve as a healing empath. If you put a shield up between yourself and those around you, you are attempting to ensure that all energy stays completely out and that your own energy stays completely in. This means that you fail to experience positive and pleasurable things to such an enjoyable degree because you are attempting to keep everything out. It also means that you struggle to interact with and enjoy your own environment. Furthermore, holding up this shield can be exhausting and can add to the many reasons why empaths often find themselves wishing that they could simply live a completely introverted life.

Another drawback of shields is that anytime you *do* engage with your environment, you produce an energetic "leak" in the shield, meaning that any energy can freely enter or exit the shield because there is now space where the shield is not being upheld. This can be a very overwhelming and frustrating experience for any empath, especially one who may just be coming into an understanding of his or her own gifts. If you have ever found yourself attempting to hold up a shield but feeling exhausted or struggling to make it actually "work," that is because, in many cases, they do not. Shields are great for moments where you truly do not want any energy coming in or going out such as in a particularly toxic environment. However, for your average outing or social experience, the shield simply won't be enough.

Creating energetic boundaries as I outlined above is truly the best way for an empath to engage in a social setting without feeling the intensely negative repercussions of the energies that are surrounding them. Through these boundaries, the empath can keep themselves feeling protected and separate from everyone else while also feeling as though they can genuinely enjoy and engage in the environment around them. Boundaries truly are the most empowering tool that you can equip yourself with as an empath as they provide all of the protection you desired from your shield without any of the energetic leaks or exhaustion.

Chapter 6: Creating a Healing Dream

Learning to control your energies and engage in energetic healing is essential for you to begin experiencing relief from your empath overwhelm right away. However, if you truly want to engage in empathic healing, you need to begin focusing on how you can create a long-term healing goal that is going to enable you to truly thrive in your life. The best way to do this is to spend time building a dream and learning how to integrate that dream into your real life.

In this chapter, we are going to explore how you can develop your healing dream so that you can truly incorporate healing and thriving into your life. This is an essential practice for anyone who wants to experience long-term healing, so make sure that you spend some time genuinely engaging in this practice. Because you are an empath, chances are that your already vivid inner world will have a great deal of fun engaging in this practice and using it as a way to create a healing experience for yourself!

The Importance of a Healing Dream

Empaths who have not yet fully embraced the path of healing and living as a confident and thriving empath may still be feeling as though they are doomed to a lifetime of experiencing overwhelm and struggling to uphold protection for themselves. This can be an exhausting and dreary outlook that can make looking forward to an enjoyable life challenging for anyone, especially someone who is sensitive and feels things so deeply.

Creating a healing dream for yourself gives you the opportunity to dream up a life that you would love living, regardless of what your empathic self currently feels. If you have dreams of being outgoing and engaged with the world around you, incorporating this into your dream is important. If you have dreams of traveling on your own, and staying mostly solo—incorporating this is also important. The real goal of your dream is identifying your authentic innermost desires and giving yourself hope that they truly can become a real experience for you.

Empaths often learn to live their entire lives around their gifts, sometimes even giving up parts of their authentic self to avoid feeling the overwhelm and exhaustion of being an empath. You want your dream to support you in learning how to live your life as *you* and incorporate being an empath into *your* life. The big difference here is that in the former experience, a person is allowing their gift to rule their life, and in the latter experience, that person is taking back control and ruling their own lives.

The purpose of your dream is to create a real visual of yourself living your best life so that you can turn that vision into your goal. This is the vision of yourself that you are going to hold onto so that you can begin engaging in healing and overcoming the troubles that have been holding you back so far. Anytime you find yourself struggling to move forward or engage in healing, this vision is going to support you in discovering what next steps need to be taken so that you can evolve in a way that includes healing your fears and taking back control.

How to Create Your Healing Dream

Creating your healing dream is as simple as sitting with your daydreams and dreaming up what you desire to have happened in your life. However, because you want this dream to remain somewhat consistent and eventually become realized, it is important that you take a few extra steps to support you in bringing this dream into your reality. Those steps include getting very specific, writing down your dream so that you can revisit it as often as you want, and releasing the outcome so that if your dream is manifested in a way that looks different from what you expected, you can still feel fulfilled by what you manifested.

Clarifying Your Vision

Clarifying your vision will ensure that you are able to truly see it and get excited about it. This also gives you something very real and specific to work towards, which is an imperative part of turning a dream into a goal. When you dream without getting specific, you leave room for many variables which makes it a challenge for you to truly aim for what you want or know if you are making progress in achieving it. Clarifying your dream requires you to spend some time thinking about the who, what, when, where, why, and how of your dream.

As you clarify your vision, look to make it as real as possible. See if you can become so clear on what your dream is that it almost feels like a memory instead of a dream. This is going to support your mind in being able to genuinely see you living your life this way, which will help you manifest your dream life. When your mind can genuinely see and feel what success looks like, it mentally prepares you for the changes you will make and the challenges you will face along the way. This is a powerful way of ensuring your success.

Writing Your Vision Down

In addition to dreaming up your vision, it can also be helpful to write it down. Writing your vision down in your journal or on a piece of paper and keeping that description nearby is a great way to allow yourself to revisit the vision on a regular basis. It also makes it feel a lot more real, as though you are writing down a goal instead of just a dream. This helps you alchemize the energy you put into your dream by transitioning it from the energy of longing for to the energy of creating.

The very act of writing down your vision also gives you the opportunity to validate yourself and the desires that you have for your life. Many people create dreams but then surround those dreams with negative beliefs or ideas that they cannot possibly bring those dreams into their reality because of any number of different reasons or excuses that they create for themselves. Writing your dream down allows you to approve of yourself and validate your desires so that you can begin generating a sense of confidence in your dream. This will help you switch your hope into faith, meaning that, you will go from hoping that it will come true to having faith that it will.

Releasing the Outcome

This may seem counterintuitive, but releasing the outcome of your dream is important, too. The reason for this is that often, the things we desire in life show up in ways that we could not have possibly expected. As you heal and evolve, your dreams are going to heal and evolve, too. This means that any dreams that you may have held onto that were the product of someone else's desires will slowly be released from your psyche and replaced with your authentic dreams and desires. It also means that as you evolve, you may find yourself being exposed to new information that calls you in a different direction from what you initially dreamed of.

Allowing yourself to release the outcome ensures that you stay subscribed to a dream that genuinely serves you and your desires. Attempting to heal yourself by forcing yourself to stay subscribed to a dream that you made in the past is only going to hold you back as this outdated dream will not support you in feeling your best at that moment. Be willing to release the outcome and allow the dream itself to evolve to truly reflect what you honestly desire in your life. Then, you will find yourself living your best life possible.

Using Your Healing Dream in a Practical Way

Aside from giving you faith and direction, your dream gives you the opportunity to begin taking practical steps towards the life you desire to live. You can use your dream to begin manifesting the next best move for you to make, to support you in feeling the way that you desire to feel, and to encourage you to stay on track at all times. When used properly, your dream is a powerful guide that can give you everything you need to move forward and live your best life.

When it comes to using your dream practically, seek to use it as the compass for how you live your life and what choices you make in your life. Look towards your dream and consult it anytime you are struggling to take action, make a change or make a choice in your life. If you are feeling stuck, pray for your dream to guide you to your next step so that you can continue making progress towards what you desire in life. If you find yourself feeling doubtful in your dream or in yourself, spend some time visualizing your desires and allowing your vision to empower you and fill you with faith and direction.

In order to maintain the practicality of your dream, make sure that you spend time allowing it to actively evolve, too. Anytime you notice that your dream no longer fully resonates with you, spend some time considering what aspects of your dream no longer resonate. This will support you in keeping your dream "up to date" so that you do not entrap yourself in an outdated dream.

Chapter 7: Healing Your Past

Empaths are often largely impacted by their past experiences in a way that can result in them having a toxic approach to life. For example, an empath who has experienced a traumatic narcissistic relationship may find themselves feeling extremely codependent and struggling to live a "normal" life because of the damage inflicted upon them by someone else. This is true for anyone who has experienced trauma, but it can be particularly challenging or damaging for empaths who have a tendency to internalize things and *feel* the trauma in a way that others may not.

In your own life, you have likely experienced many larger and smaller traumas that have led to you feeling as though you are in need of healing. As an empath, you have likely found yourself being exposed to more traumatic experiences or events than others who are not considered empaths. This is because the internalization of energy and emotions can feel traumatic, leading to experiences that may be "normal" for others feeling traumatic to empaths. It is also because other people tend to recognize that empaths are vulnerable and either consciously or subconsciously takes advantage of the empath. As an empath, you are more vulnerable to negative experiences such as those including narcissists and energy vampires.

Healing your past experiences is going to allow you to end the cycle of other people taking control over you and give you the opportunity to take control over yourself once again. When you combine the healing of your past with the process of taking control over your own energy, you create the opportunity for you to become a truly powerful person. Your capacity to feel confident and strong in yourself while also feeling tender and compassionate towards others in a way that is not damaging unto yourself is a mix that will allow you to heal the collective without draining yourself in order to do it.

Identifying Your Life Lessons

One way that you can significantly improve your healing experience is through identifying your life lessons. Life lessons are the lessons that take root early on in our childhood and show up time and again through patterns that we experience in our lives. Each person has their own unique life lessons to be learned, though you may find that your life lessons overlap with other people's lessons.

Identifying your life lessons is going to support you in learning these lessons and integrating them into your life so that you can begin living with a more wholesome and controlled approach to life. It is also going to help you understand why certain energy types may impact you more than others, thus causing your empathic gifts to feel overburdened when you are out and about. Anytime you experience the energy of someone who triggers your life lesson, it will leave a lasting impact that is far greater than any of the other energies that you experience. Left unmanaged, these energies can become extremely overwhelming and frustrating to deal with.

The easiest way to begin identifying what your life lessons might be is to look back through your lifetime of experiences and consider what patterns you see in the traumatic or challenging experiences that you have. Identifying the patterns that you experience in your life will help you begin to uncover what it is that you may need to learn. It is important to understand that truly grasping what that lesson is, will take more time and self-awareness, as these lessons are often buried in our subconscious mind until we bring them forward to be addressed, assessed, and integrated.

Once you have a general sense of what these patterns are, take them for their face value and consider what their lessons may be. For example, if you have consistently been surrounded by narcissists in your past, your experience may be to learn how to spot narcissists and protect yourself against them. This is a great opportunity to start integrating your life lessons and overcoming these challenges so that you can take control over your life once again. However, realizing that life lessons are not always obvious, you need to continue looking into this trigger or lesson to see how specific you can get. Ask yourself questions such as "how am I attracting these narcissists?" "How may I be struggling to protect myself against this?" or "why am I vulnerable in this situation?" can support you in learning more about your unique circumstances. You may discover that the underlying lesson is that you need to be more compassionate toward yourself and your own needs, or that you need to stop trying to superimpose in other people's lives and "save them" from themselves.

Identifying these life lessons and really getting into the root of what they are, why they are there, and how they can be learned is going to support you in feeling a stronger sense of control in your life. Rather than feeling deeply triggered by something and not entirely knowing why or feeling haunted by a particular type of energy in your life, you can begin to take control and integrate this lesson so that you are no longer bothered by these triggers or energies. As an empath, having this type of self-awareness and personal control is life-changing in that it allows you to stop feeling so overburdened by the energies around you. Healing your past and understanding your experiences are great ways to experience confidence in yourself and your ability to live a better life.

How You Can Heal Your Past

Your life lessons have been deeply ingrained in your past and have likely impacted your life in a massive way. For some empaths, their life lessons can result in their personality changing completely until they are able to integrate the lessons and learn from them. For example, an empath who was extroverted as a child but endured many lessons echoing the same purpose may find themselves overwhelmed and anxious, thus leading to them living life as an introvert to avoid the pain. Healing your past is imperative as it will support you in accessing your authentic self so that you can stop living as a victim of your past and your empathic gifts.

Healing your past can be done in many ways, though it usually requires a healthy mixture of approaches to ensure that you are experiencing thorough healing. It can also take a fair bit of time as you are going to be diving into previous experiences of trauma, discomfort, pain, and suffering as a way to relieve this pain and move forward in your life. It is usually best to do this alongside someone who can offer you compassionate support without interrupting your healing process. Ideally, this should be a therapist who can support you through practices such as talk therapy, although a trusted friend would do well in many cases, too.

Below I have listed five practices that you can begin using to release and heal from these past hurts.

Make the Decision to Let It Go

Before you can truly heal from anything, you need to make the decision that you are ready to let it go. Getting into the mindset of letting things go allows you to shift from the position of holding onto your pain so that you can truly move on. Often, we desire to let something go from our past but we are unable or unwilling to turn that desire into a decision so that we can truly do so. What ends up happening is that, even though we desire to move on, we sit with that pain and continue to see ourselves as victims of the experiences that we had. In the end, the only person who continues suffering is ourselves.

To make the decision, you simply need to agree with yourself that you are ready to truly let go of the experience you had. This does not mean that the experience is in any way lessened, invalidated, or deemed as "ok" but instead, it means that you are willing to accept it for what it is and move forward knowing that it cannot be changed. In this acceptance and willingness, you find the opportunity to begin performing true healing on yourself and in your life.

Express Your Pain

Now that you have made the decision to let your pain go, you need to make the effort to truly express your pain. If you attempt to let something go without genuinely expressing the pain you have felt, you are going to find yourself struggling to truly let it go because there are still many repressed emotions attached to that experience. Allowing yourself to feel through the pain and express it in a productive way helps you move the energy out of yourself so that you can continue down your path of healing.

As an empath, this is your essential step to ensuring that you no longer hold onto so many different overwhelming energies in your energy body. By releasing these energies, you give yourself the opportunity to start from a clean slate. You will no longer feel overwhelmed so quickly and easily because you will not be attempting to take on more energies on top of the all of the ones you are already holding on to.

Take Responsibility

In choosing to let go of something, you need to take responsibility for your experience. This means that you are no longer choosing to stay in the victim mentality where you blame the other person because you are now taking responsibility for your life and your experiences. This does not mean that you take the blame of someone else's wrongdoings or make their consequences your own. Instead, it means that you are choosing to take responsibility for the process of healing and letting go of what they have done to you.

This very process of taking responsibility moves you out of the victim mentality and supports you in taking control over your life.

Empaths have a strong tendency of living in the victim mentality when they have yet to take control over themselves and their energy which can often lead to the belief that being an empath is a curse. This stems from not knowing how to take responsibility for themselves and their experiences. In doing so, you allow yourself to experience liberation from your difficult experiences so that you can begin experiencing a better life.

Focus On the Present

After you have chosen to let go, expressed all of your emotions, and taken responsibility for yourself and your choices, you have completed everything you need to do regarding the past. Now, you need to begin focusing on the present and how you can make your current life better. This is a wonderful opportunity for you to begin considering the consequences of your painful experience and how it has been shaping your life since it happened. You can also look into your empathic gifts and consider how your experience may be causing you to experience certain emotions stronger than others when it comes to emotionally and energetically taking over other people's experiences. In many cases, you will find that the emotions you tend to be hijacked by the most are directly related to previous painful experiences you have had in your own life.

As you choose to live in the present, consider how you can begin living your life in a more authentic and fulfilling manner. Seek the opportunity to discover how you can continue overcoming the repercussions of your previous pains so that you can live in a way that genuinely feels good for you. Choose to continually live in the light of healing. Any time you experience something that would have triggered you as a result of that past experience, make the conscious effort to let go and move forward in your life in that very moment.

Practice Forgiveness

The final step of healing is to forgive yourself and forgive anyone who has hurt you in your past. Forgiveness is your opportunity to truly take back control in your present and stop your past self and people from your past from hurting you any further. You may find that, in some cases, forgiveness requires a regular recommitment in order for you to truly stay in forgiveness with yourself and others. It is important that you honor the process of forgiveness no matter how it looks for you so that you can continue feeling freedom from your previous pains.

As an empath, forgiveness truly is a liberating experience. When you forgive, you alchemize the painful energy of victim consciousness and lift yourself into a state of resuming control over yourself and your life. This is the step where you actually clear out the residual energy of the past so that you do not feel as though you are constantly attempting to approach life from a cup that is already overflowing with stress and overwhelm. Instead, you can approach life with the ability to see things clearly and with freedom from your past.

Chapter 8: Healing Your Inner Child

Even though you have already begun taking action toward healing your past, there is a further action that needs to be done if you are going to experience true and complete healing in your life. As an empath, an important part of healing is addressing your inner child and healing this part of yourself, too. While healing your past will contribute to the healing of your inner child, there are further actions that should be taken to support your inner child in healing completely.

Your inner child is the part of yourself that still sees the past as if they were living in the past, and not through your more experienced and understanding eyes now. That is why it needs to be healed independently of your past healing that is being completed as an adult. For many empaths, healing the inner child is an incredibly liberating experience that supports them in truly and completely feeling free of their past troubles. This is the opportunity to fully overcome that small inner voice that keeps crying "danger" every time you see a trigger that even remotely reflects an example you have had in the past. By healing your inner child, you allow yourself to stop feeling quite so on edge every time you go out for a social event or find yourself in a public space. When your inner child is healed, it no longer feels so worried and fearful of the world around it which allows you to approach life through a more calmed state. As a result, addressing and dealing with any energy you may face in your life becomes a lot easier.

Healing your inner child is important for anyone who desires complete healing in their lives, but it is especially important for empaths. Since you have been highly sensitive all your life, chances are that you have plenty of memories you can recall where you felt the repercussions of your sensitivities. The way people talked to you, the energy they had when they talked to you, and even the energy of the environments you frequented would all have left lasting imprints on your mind as you were growing up. This means that you have even more healing to consider as compared to the average person who did not experience heightened levels of sensitivities their entire life.

How to Access Your Inner Child

The first step in healing your inner child is actually accessing your inner child so that you can begin sharing communications with this part of yourself. You can think of your inner child as that small voice inside of you that still thinks, talks, and behaves like a child despite the fact that you are now an adult. For example, when you feel angry and an inner part of you begins to experience the feelings of a temper tantrum even though your adult self-recognizes that a temper tantrum is not a valid or productive response to your anger. This inner part of you that still wants to respond to situations in a more emotional and less rational sense reflects your inner child.

Accessing your inner child requires you to truly take the time to recognize that it exists and that it both needs and wants to be acknowledged. Allowing yourself to become aware of this need and to recognize it as a part of yourself that is valid and important supports you in giving your inner child the safe space it needs to emerge into. Then, you need to begin speaking to your inner child. Speaking to your inner child allows you to give it the attention it requires while also gaining understanding from it about why it is feeling and behaving the way it is. This is the very information that you will use to work towards healing so that you can begin feeling emotional freedom and stop feeling so overwhelmed by your sensitivity.

Some people who are more drawn into using physical objects or their environment as a way to engage in mental and spiritual practices may find that accessing their inner child is easier if they have something from their childhood. For example, holding a picture of your younger self or sitting with your childhood teddy bear may help stimulate your inner child and encourage him or her to come out and spend some time sharing with you. If you do not have any belongings from your childhood, you can always gather an object that resembles something you had in childhood.

Once you have acknowledged and recognized that energy within you, you can begin talking to your inner child and asking it questions. Some great questions to start off with include "How are you?" or "What would you like me to know right now?" This encourages this part of your psyche to begin engaging with you and sharing information about how it may be feeling in response to the world around it. For empaths, this part of yourself likely experiences a lot of fear and anxiety around the experiences that you have as an adult. Bringing it to the forefront and acknowledging it is a powerful way to start the healing process so that your inner child can stop feeling traumatized by the world around you.

How to Gain Your Inner Child's Trust

Believe it or not, you do have to gain the trust of your inner child if you want to have the opportunity to fully embrace the process of healing your inner child. Many empaths find that their inner child experiences feelings of betrayal, abandonment, neglect, or even simply being forgotten about. This is because most people don't realize that their inner child still exists and that it still needs support in understanding and overcoming challenges in life. Anytime you endure or embrace a new challenge in life, your inner child will still respond in the very same way that your childhood-self did. Despite the evolution you have endured, you still have an inner part of you that struggles with seeing, understanding, and responding to the world around you. This part of you wants to be loved, respected, cherished, and appreciated by those around you and by yourself. It also wants to have you show it affection and be compassionate and tender towards it, oftentimes reflecting something that you may have never fully experienced as a child.

In life, our inner child often feels abandoned and neglected when it is not given the tender compassion and love that it needs during those moments of sensitivity, especially as an empath. As an adult, your inner child will still naturally respond with this feeling right away even if you do not acknowledge it or even become aware of it. For this reason, your inner child has now grown to see you as untrustworthy, too. So, gaining the trust of your inner child is important.

As an empath, chances are your inner child is feeling wounded because it continues to worry that it is "too sensitive" or "taking things too seriously." This part of you still stings every time someone tells you that you need to grow a thicker skin or recognizes a joke when you hear one even if it doesn't sound funny to you. Despite you now having a better awareness around these experiences or even having a greater sense of compassion towards yourself and your sensitivity, your inner child still longs for that tenderness and compassion.

You can gain the trust of your inner child by showing it that you now recognize it still exists and that you are willing to acknowledge it and stay aware of it. By showing your inner child that you did not forget about them but rather that you did not realize they were still there, you can ask your inner child for forgiveness and then work towards gaining their trust. In doing so, you bring more comfort to your inner child. Reassure your inner childhood self that you are there for them (yourself) now and that you want to listen to them, see them, and support them in their experiences. You need to be extremely tender and gentle with yourself while also remaining consistent and devoted so that your inner child can see that you are serious about supporting it.

If your inner child has been repressed for a long time, the process of gaining its trust and being able to fully access it and listen to it may take some time. Be patient with yourself and continue to practice listening to your inner child so that you can show it that you are trustworthy. The more you practice this step, the more your inner child will open up to you and share its feelings and the experiences it is holding onto. This is going to help you get a deep understanding of your own emotions and why you may be so sensitive to certain experiences as opposed to others or even more sensitive to all experiences in general.

How to Heal Your Inner Child

Once you have accessed and gained the trust of your inner child, you can begin working towards healing it. The best way to begin healing your inner child is to allow yourself to express the emotions that are being felt by your inner child. Allow all of these feelings that you are experiencing during these conversations to rise to the surface and be expressed in a way that is complete and healthy. If you are experiencing fear, allow yourself to shake it out. If you feel like crying because you are feeling sadness or shame, let that come out, too. Use this opportunity to feel and release any emotion that wants to rise to the surface and be felt.

When you express the emotions that your inner child has not had the opportunity to fully express, you allow yourself to release the energy that is being entrapped by that memory or experience. This allows you to completely release that inner "bottle" that has been filling up over the years and restore a state of peace and calm inside of you.

As you release these emotions, you may feel a sense of worry in regards to the intensity of the emotions that come up. You might find yourself feeling worried that these emotions will become overpowering or that you will not be able to control them. Trust that this is not the case and that you will still be able to experience full control over your emotions even as they come out. That fear belongs to your inner child and it is worried that it will lose control as it was told that losing control was wrong. You are now an adult who is capable of staying in control while expressing your emotions so you do not need to worry about this experience. Simply let the fear be expressed and then move on to experiencing your other emotions as well. This way, you can experience a complete release of your emotions and you can release the incredible amounts of energy attached to those emotions.

Chances are that your inner child will only express a few things at a time. After all, you were a child for many years, so there are many years of experiences that may need to be recognized and expressed. As you continue working with this practice you will find yourself feeling a greater sense of release each time. Over time, you may find that your inner child is contented and that you no longer have the need to engage in such healing practices. By the time this happens, you should find that your ability to process life as an empath is much easier as well, since you now experience greater control over yourself, your energies, and your emotions.

Chapter 9: Healing Your Current Self

The next thing that you need to heal as an empath involves your current self. Healing your current self is an opportunity for you to release anything that may be causing energetic or emotional turmoil in your life right now so that you can maximize your ability to truly enjoy life. For the most part, healing your current self requires you to consider what your current state of wellbeing is and begin healing that version of yourself. Healing your past and inner child will support you in feeling a release from the attachments that have been holding you in this state, but healing your current self will allow you to fully release the symptoms that were caused by your past. For empaths, healing the current self, allows them to begin experiencing a greater sense of self-confidence and self-esteem so that they can begin enjoying life from a more intentional and empowered point of view.

In this chapter, we are going to explore how healing your current self can improve your life and how you can use your improved self-esteem and self-confidence to experience a better life as an empath. Even if you are someone who already considers their self-esteem and self-confidence to be fairly high, working on this healing practice will ensure that you are using this strong sense of self to support your inner empath in the best ways possible.

Identifying What Needs Healing

Before you can begin healing your current self, you first need to consider what may be wrong. Looking into your past makes seeing trauma or challenges easy as you can now see how they impacted your life at the time. Looking at your current life and trying to consider what may be "going wrong" can feel more challenging because these are the behaviors, thoughts, and experiences that you are actively engaging in.

To identify what may need to be healed, spend some time with your journal writing down the things about your current life that you wish were different or improved. Consider everything from the way you communicate with others and yourself to the way you approach various situations in your life. All of these experiences contain massive amounts of energy which can impact your empathic self and leave you feeling vulnerable, overdrawn, or overburdened by the world around you. If left untouched, they can result in you living your life according to your gift rather than using your gift to support you in living a better life.

As you are addressing what needs to be healed, do not be afraid to consider parts of yourself that were caused by past experiences, even if you have already intentionally worked towards healing these past experiences. Many times, our past experiences result in current problems that also need to be addressed. Just because you healed the memory of the pain does not mean that the symptoms are not still lingering in your behavior, thoughts, and attitude at this time. Addressing the current self that needs healing too will support you in fully healing from past experiences so that you can move forward and begin living a better life altogether, completely free of any attachments to the past.

It is likely that you will find many things that need to be addressed or healed to some degree. This will not end, either. Healing is an ongoing process that will regularly need to be addressed and worked on to ensure that you are always staying at your peak energy. The best way to ensure that you are always identifying aspects of yourself that can be healed is through regular self-reflection and journaling. This will support you in staying self-aware and remaining fully committed to your healing practice.

The Importance of Self-Awareness

If you are not already a self-aware person, self-healing can be a fairly challenging process. Being able to heal yourself requires you to be able to actually look into yourself and notice the parts of yourself that can be healing. As an empath, self-awareness tends to be something that comes naturally and will inevitably support you in your healing journey. However, you may also find that if you are living in the archetype of the "cursed" empathy, you have repressed your feelings and your sense of self for quite a long time. Some empaths even report feeling out of body experiences or experiences of dissociation as a way to detach from the painful experiences of being an empath. In these circumstances, self-awareness may be more challenging for you to achieve.

If you are not already living in a state of self-awareness, you are going to want to begin practicing so that you can have a stronger understanding of yourself and your needs. The best way to begin practicing self-awareness is to regularly check in and ask yourself how you are doing and if there is anything that you need. Asking yourself questions like this require you to truly check in with your feelings, thoughts, and needs and then follow through on taking care of yourself. This establishes a strong relationship between you and yourself that supports you in feeling worthy of your own time and attention. Like with the inner child healings, you may find that you need to work towards gaining your own trust in order to fully embrace the art of self-awareness. Continue showing yourself compassion and tenderness and you will likely find that self-awareness seems to come naturally from this growing relationship that you share with yourself.

Releasing the Final Ties of the Past

Now that you have brought your desire for healing into your current state of awareness, you can begin the process of truly healing these experiences that you have been having. Since all of your current troubles will have been cultivated by your previous traumas, this requires you to finally release all of your current ties to the past. The best way to envision this process is to consider the experience as the removal of a weed. Healing your past and inner child allowed you to heal the roots of the problem. Now, you need to remove the rest of the plant that grew off of those roots to produce the person that you are today.

Releasing the final ties to your past does not actually require your past in any significant manner. While having an idea of why you behave the way you do can support you in having a greater sense of understanding, it is not actually necessary. What is necessary is that you address each part of yourself that needs healing and you begin to understand why it is no longer serving you and how it may be alchemized to serve you better. For example, if you find that you have a tendency to become overwhelmed around certain energies even though you have to face them on a regular basis, you may set the intention to heal your response around these energies. In addition to setting this intention, you can also determine how you would like to behave instead.

Using your healing dream is a great way to support you in healing your current self. Through your healing dream, you can "see" the way you would prefer to behave and begin visualizing yourself actually behaving in this manner. This visualization will help you as you gradually work towards swapping out your current mannerisms with new ones that will support you in manifesting your healing dream into reality. The process of changing these now-outdated behaviors is the final tie of the past that you will officially cut loose. Following this change, you will feel as though you are fully liberated from that experience that once held you in a state of energetic and emotional turmoil. This liberation will allow you to feel more confident in yourself and in your ability to assert your boundaries, including your energetic boundaries so that you can take back control over your life and stop feeling as though you are being victimized by your empathic gifts.

Incorporating Self-Healing On a Regular Basis

It is important that you truly understand that healing is an ongoing experience. You will never fully be "healed" because there will always be more that can be addressed, assessed, and improved upon. If you truly want to embrace healing, you need to be willing to embrace the full journey that comes along with it, no matter how long or enduring it may be. Some parts of the process may be challenging, painful, or simply frustrating. Other parts may feel as though you have waited far too long for the healing itself and you are genuinely excited to overcome your troubles and begin living a better life. In the end, the version of you that has experienced greater amounts of healing will sincerely appreciate your efforts.

Incorporating your healing into your regular routine is a requirement if you want to truly embrace a healing journey. The best way to do this is through regular self-reflection, journaling, and dreaming. The more you recognize parts of yourself that are unhealed and dream up what it would be like for them to be healed, the easier it will be for you to visualize and then manifest yourself living your best life possible. As an empath, using healing energy in this way will provide you with great liberation from the overwhelm that sensitivity can bring your way.

Chapter 10: Social Healing Practices

Empaths are rarely fully appreciated and accepted by society in our current world because society has a tendency to be a lot harsher in its energy than empaths can handle. As an empath in a society, experiencing and expressing your sensitive side may not always be well-received. This can lead to you feeling as though you are not welcome in the society. This can further stimulate your inner feelings of abandonment and neglect and can result in you experiencing an inner emotional trauma from the "broken" relationship between yourself and others in general.

Learning how to heal your social experiences can support you in engaging in social experiences on a greater level so that you can begin enjoying the public or experiences that require you to go out in the public. In this chapter, we are going to explore how you can heal that feeling of being an outcast that is frowned upon by society so that you can begin enjoying a better life and feeling genuinely fulfilled in every way possible. Whether you are an introverted or an extroverted empath does not matter, these practices will support your healing all the same.

Taking Responsibility for Yourself

The first step in having better social experiences is taking responsibility for yourself. Learning how to take responsibility for your energies and your experience supports you in staying clear of the victim mentality. This will keep you from feeling as though you are constantly being attacked any time you go in public because you will be able to prevent these feelings of energetic attack. When you realize that society does not dislike you and that you are absolutely welcomed into the world as it is, it becomes a lot easier for you to stop taking everything quite so personally. That way, you can stop feeling as though everyone else's energies belong to you and that you have to assume responsibility for them.

As an empath, one of the worst beliefs that you can possibly hold is that you are responsible for any energies or emotions that come into your space. This is not true. You are only responsible for your own energies and emotions. If they are being impacted or influenced by someone else's energies or emotions, it is your responsibility to recognize that and adjust your approach to the situation to avoid having an unwanted energetic or emotional experience. When you take responsibility for yourself, it becomes a lot easier to stop taking responsibility for other people which will support you in enforcing your energetic boundaries so that you no longer take on emotions or energies that are not yours.

Healing the "Sponge" Belief

An unfortunate belief that circulates the empath circle is that empaths are "sponges" that constantly "sop up" other people's emotions and energies. This is certainly what it can feel like when you are not actively taking care of yourself and your energies but once you start to, this symptom goes away, meaning that you are not doomed to feeling like a sponge forever. Believing that you are always going to be a sponge that constantly absorbs the energies and emotions of other people can feel extremely easy to believe considering that you have felt it in the past *and* that you are an empath so your feeling is reinforced by others. However, when you choose to take responsibility for yourself and your energies and you begin practicing energetic boundaries, it becomes a lot easier for you to stop absorbing everyone else's energies.

It is important that you begin choosing to foster a new belief as soon as possible to avoid allowing this belief to continue enforcing your feelings of absorption. The more you say this belief out loud, the more you reinforce that your boundaries are meaningless because energy will simply come through anyway. In other words, you are effectively rendering your boundaries meaningless because you are singlehandedly ignoring them and allowing yourself to feel unwanted energies. You need to take responsibility *and* discard the belief that anyone that is not you has any control over your energies whatsoever.

Healing Your Relationship with the Society

As you begin to take responsibility for yourself, you also need to take responsibility for your relationship with society. Chances are that the part of you that still lives in fear and shame around society is your inner child. This means that you will likely have some healing to do with your inner child around the topic of society and other people. In addition to that, you need to consider your adult self and how you currently feel about society. If your feelings about society are poor, such as you believe that everyone is too harsh and that no one appreciates or understands you, you are going to reinforce this negative belief and struggle in society no matter what.

If you choose to adjust your beliefs and see society as a beautiful opportunity to connect with other people and, maybe, meet people who are sensitive like yourself, then suddenly, society becomes a lot less scary and a lot more enjoyable. When you adjust your beliefs in this way, you allow yourself to heal from those inner feelings associated with being an outcast or someone who was too weak for society.

In healing your relationship with the society, you give yourself back your freedom. Whether you like it or not, you live as a part of a society and living at odds with the world is never going to support you in feeling any better. If anything, it will leave you feeling exceptionally vulnerable to the energy of those around you because you will constantly find yourself focusing on the judgmental, rude, and hurtful energies of others. As a result, your empathic self will feel extremely overwhelmed every time you go out in public. If, however, you see society as an opportunity or as a simple fact of life, suddenly, these energies will not be so intimidating or fearsome to you and you will be able to enjoy society with a greater sense of ease.

Allowing Yourself to Have Fun

Empaths often struggle to have fun in ways that are not directly associated with being alone or doing something quiet and withdrawn. While there is nothing wrong with being an introvert or preferring reading and movies over going out and being with a group of people, it is not effective if you are the type of person who only chooses books or movies because of your fear of society. If the constant nagging worry of going out and enjoying yourself keeps you from actually going out and doing it, then you need to practice learning how to completely detach from the world around you so that you can let loose and just have fun. This may seem impossible, but it is actually entirely possible and can make your life significantly better.

Allowing yourself to have fun ultimately requires a commitment from you to yourself. In that commitment, you need to commit to allowing yourself to not worry about the energies or emotions of those around you in a way that results in you feeling overwhelmed or responsible for their experience. While you can certainly acknowledge their energies or emotions, allow yourself permission to completely detach from them so that you can stop feeling them as your own. Instead, commit to simply enjoying yourself and enjoying the world around you without feeling quite so overwhelmed and exhausted from these experiences.

At first, making this commitment may seem downright impossible. It may even seem harsh to detach because you might worry that detaching will prevent you from feeling any level of emotion, including empathy. This is not the case. Detaching in a healthy manner is going to allow you to detach from feeling *personally responsible* for someone else. You will still be able to experience and express empathy, amongst other emotions, but you will not feel such a nagging and overwhelming need to engage in experiences that do not belong to you. It may benefit you to begin practicing this type of detachment in environments that are not quite so overwhelming at first so that you can get the hang of it. As you do, continue increasing the intensity of your environment as much as you would like, allowing yourself to fully embrace your detachment at each "level" until you feel comfortable and ready to move up. Doing it at your own pace will help you feel more confident in your control over yourself and your ability to detach from the intense energies around you.

Advocating For Yourself When You Need To

Being an advocate for yourself is essential if you want to practice being more involved in society as an empath. As your own personal advocate, you will be responsible for paying attention to your needs and your desires any time you are out and about in public. This is a part of taking responsibility for yourself, but it is an essential component that truly does require its own independent attention.

In being an advocate for yourself, you need to be willing to not only identify your needs and desires but also ensure that they are met. For example, if you are feeling particularly overwhelmed by your environment, you need to speak up for yourself about your need to go step outside for a few minutes or to excuse yourself from the event so that you can retreat to a more relaxed environment. No matter what your need is, it is never too big or too small to be addressed. It is also never too unreasonable to be requested, especially when it is a need. If you are spending time with anyone who does not honor your right to express your needs and actively fulfill them, you need to begin spending time around people who are more considerate over you and your desires. Still, regardless of who you are around or what attitude they may have, you are responsible for ensuring that your own needs are being met. You must make sure that you are advocating for yourself and your needs at all times so that you can stay in trust with yourself and feel more confident in your outings.

Conclusion

Congratulations on completing "Empath!"

I hope that by reading this book, you were able to discover more about yourself and experience a greater sense of self-awareness through the explanations that I offered. By understanding yourself to a greater degree, you give yourself the power that you need to begin taking control in your own life and experiencing a greater quality of life overall. You will no longer feel as though you are living at the mercy of those around you the more you practice taking control over your life.

As an empath, you will find yourself picking up on energies that other people may not even realize that they have. Experiencing these energies when the person responsible for the energies is not even willing to experience them is a burden that no one needs to take. In order to live your best life, you need to learn to take responsibility for yourself and heal the parts of you that have led you to believe otherwise. By healing these parts of yourself, you allow yourself to empty out the "reserve" of unhealed energies that live inside of you, so that you can approach life from a greater sense of personal power and confidence. Through that, you will access your best life.

After you finish reading this book, it is important that you continue practicing mastering your gift of being an empath. The more you engage in healing and taking back your power while also reinforcing personal energetic boundaries, the easier it will be for you to continue mastering your gift. Then, you can step into your true calling of being a healer, teacher, caretaker or otherwise. When you are able to embrace this calling from a place of power, you will begin to discover ways that your empathic gift can genuinely help you rather than hinder you from experiencing a complete success. Any empath who attempts to embrace their true calling without first mastering the gift of being an empath will likely find themselves quickly feeling burnt out from following their passion. This can lead to a myriad of new problems, including the need to experience further healing in their lives specifically around their passions. To avoid burnout and exhaustion, master the art of being an empath first and embrace your true calling second.

Lastly, if you enjoyed this book, I ask that you please take the time to honestly review it on Amazon Kindle. Your feedback would be greatly appreciated.

Thank you!

Made in United States
North Haven, CT
31 January 2023